HOW TO COUNT CARB FOR BETTER BLOOD SUGAR CONTROL

Conquer your blood sugar swing permanently and live a healthier, happier you

INTRODUCTION

Farewell, Blood Sugar Rollercoaster. Hello, Empowered You!

Have you ever felt as if your blood sugar was the conductor of your life's orchestra, controlling your energy levels, food choices, and even your mood? You are not alone. Millions of people suffer from blood sugar fluctuations, a never-ending cycle of highs and lows that makes them feel out of control. Imagine a society in which food becomes an ally rather than an enemy. A world in which you understand what fuels your body and how to navigate a world full of delectable options without worrying about blood sugar spikes or crashes. This book is your ticket to that world, your guide to discovering the secret weapon in blood sugar management: carb counting.

Forget rigid diets and tedious calorie counting. Carb counting is a wonderful tool that provides you with knowledge rather than constraints. It's about understanding how carbohydrates affect your body and how to use that information to your advantage. Consider it a breakthrough in reading the secret language on food labels, transforming complicated verbiage into simple health guidelines.

This book is more than just a list of numbers and calculations. It's a voyage of personal discovery and empowerment. We'll look at the science of blood sugar clearly and interestingly, dispelling myths and misconceptions along the way. We'll explore the intriguing world of carbs, learning to distinguish between the good, the bad, and the sly ones that hide in plain sight.

Most importantly, we will turn all of this information into actionable plans. You'll learn to:

Become a Food Label Detective: Decode nutrition data panels with greater confidence, discover hidden carbs, make smart grocery store purchases, and make other purchasing decisions.

Create a personalized carb budget. Set realistic goals depending on your activity level and health objectives.

Master the art of food planning. Create delicious, carb-conscious meals for all occasions, including breakfast, dinner, and everything in between.

Navigate the Restaurant Jungle: De-mystify dining out and make healthy, delicious choices without jeopardizing your blood sugar goals.

Adopt a holistic approach: Discover the benefits of sleep, stress management, and self-care in controlling your blood sugar.

So let go of your fear and frustration. Let us go on this trip together. With this book as your guide and a little practice, you'll go from being a passenger on the blood sugar rollercoaster to a confident driver, navigating your way to optimal health and happiness. Are you ready to take control of your blood sugar and explore a world of delectable possibilities? Let us begin!

Chapter 1

The Blood Sugar Blues

How I Reclaimed My Energy

Imagine this: You're in the middle of a work presentation, passionately and confidently setting forth your amazing proposal. Suddenly, a rush of exhaustion hits you. Your hands begin to tremble, your thoughts get hazy, and that lovely morning cappuccino you promised would not raise your blood sugar now seems like a distant memory. This wasn't just an ordinary afternoon slump; it was a typical case of the "Blood Sugar Blues," a word I sadly became intimately familiar with during my adventure with fluctuating blood sugar.

For years, I fought an invisible evil within. My energy levels were erratic, surging after meals only to sink an hour later, leaving me exhausted and irritated. These crashes were more than just inconvenient; they affected every part of my existence. The afternoon slump became a regular visitor, hurting job productivity and making me want to nap rather than go to the gym.

What is the worst part? The unpredictability. There was no rhyme or reason for the crashes. An apparently nutritious salad would occasionally cause a drop, yet a single piece of fruit could keep me energized for hours. I painstakingly logged my meals, researched healthy eating, and even took numerous supplements in the desperate goal of regaining some sense of control. However, the blood sugar rollercoaster resumed its unrelenting trip.

It wasn't just physical, either. The continual worry over my blood sugar levels adds a layer of mental stress to my daily activities. Social outings became a cause of dread for me: would I have the energy to participate? Could I trust the restaurant to provide healthy selections that would not cause me to crash? Even simple things like grocery shopping became difficult, with interpreting labels and counting carbs becoming a daily mental fight.

Now, as a healthcare worker, I witness other patients dealing with identical issues. Their stories are incredibly moving—the frustration, the dread, the sense of being held captive by their bodies. But there's good news: it doesn't have to be this way. There is a way to reclaim control, understand what fuels your body, and navigate the world of food with confidence. In this book, we'll go on that trip together, discovering the intriguing world of blood sugar and the powerful instrument that altered my life: carb counting.

This isn't just another stringent diet regimen. Carb counting is an approach to understanding the code on food labels and making informed decisions. It's about arming oneself with knowledge and applying it to create a tailored approach to blood sugar management.

The ongoing battle with changing blood sugar left me searching for answers. I perused research papers, spoke with other healthcare experts, and eventually discovered a concept that proved my saving grace: blood sugar regulation. It looked simple enough: keep your blood sugar in a healthy range, and the crazy fluctuations would subside. But the question remained: what was producing the variations in the first place?

The culprit, I quickly realized, was a familiar foe: carbs. Carbohydrates are the body's major source of energy; they are broken down into glucose (sugar) and taken into the bloodstream. The difficulty arises when this process occurs too quickly, causing a surge in blood sugar. Consider how a sudden rainstorm would overburden a drainage system. Your body secretes insulin, a hormone that works as a key, unlocking cells and allowing glucose to enter for energy synthesis.

However, the body does not always create enough insulin, and cells might become resistant to its actions. This can result in an accumulation of glucose in the bloodstream, known as hyperglycemia. The initial energy rush can be misleading. However, when the body struggles to manage the excess sugar, the inevitable fall occurs exhaustion, cognitive fog, and a strong need for another sugar fix to re-energize.

This newly discovered understanding proved to be a turning point. I began paying close attention to how certain foods influenced my blood sugar. For example, a bagel for breakfast may provide a momentary energy boost, followed by a mid-morning slump. On the other hand, a breakfast high in protein and healthy fats, combined with a moderate amount of complex carbs, kept me energized for longer.

These personal tests were the foundation for my carb-counting adventure. Understanding how different carbohydrates affected my blood sugar allowed me to make more informed decisions. The goal was balance and control, not elimination. Imagine a world where you can eat great food without worrying about a blood sugar drop. Imagine waking up rejuvenated and ready to face the day. Imagine a life free of the anxiety and frustration caused by unpredictable blood sugar variations. This is the world that welcomes you on the other side of the blood sugar lows.

My journey with carb counting was not a straight line to success. Sometimes I misjudged carbs or consumed a sugary treat, resulting in the typical crash. But with each event, I learned and adjusted. I improved my carb-counting skills, but more importantly, I gained a better understanding of my body's response to certain foods.

Power of Self-Discovery

Carb counting became a method of self-discovery. It wasn't just about numbers on a chart; it was about becoming an expert on my health. I discovered which foods offered prolonged energy, which caused crashes, and how to manage social situations without jeopardizing my health goals.

Carb counting was a major change, but it was not the only option. A balanced diet rich in fruits, vegetables, whole grains, and lean meats became a top concern. I also learned the value of getting adequate quality sleep, reducing stress through techniques such as meditation, and including regular exercise in my routine.

The impact extended beyond physical health. A sense of empowerment replaced the continual concern over blood sugar levels. I felt in control of my health and energy levels, which enabled me to fully engage in life's adventures. Social outings became a source of joy rather than dread. Meal preparation has become an interesting exploration of new healthy recipes.

If you're experiencing blood sugar blues, remember that you're not alone. But there is hope. This book is your guide to a better, happier you. In the next chapters, we'll look at the science underlying blood sugar, the many types of carbs and their effects on your body, and give you the tools you need to take control. We'll also dispel common carb myths and misconceptions, as well as present a step-by-step roadmap to carb counting success.

This path may take some effort, but the benefits are immeasurable: a life free of blood sugar fluctuations, a revitalized sense of energy, and the ability to live life to the fullest. Are you ready to let go of the blood sugar blues and embrace a brighter, healthier future? Let us begin!

Chapter 2

Inside the Blood Sugar Machine

Demystifying the Sweet Symphony

Consider your body to be a vibrant metropolis that is continually alive with action. To keep this metropolis running, its inhabitants (your cells) require a constant source of energy, which is where blood sugar comes in. Blood sugar, commonly known as glucose, is the fuel that powers your cells, allowing you to think effectively, move your muscles, and keep your entire body functioning properly.

The Sweet Delivery System

Here's how the energy supply system works:

The Food Chain: The journey begins with what you consume. Carbohydrates, the primary source of blood sugar, are degraded into smaller molecules during digestion. Imagine deconstructing a train into separate cars. These smaller molecules, primarily simple carbohydrates such as glucose, are then taken into your bloodstream via the intestines.

The Insulin Highway: Once in your bloodstream, glucose behaves like cars on a highway, ready to transport fuel to your cells. This is when insulin, a major actor, enters the picture. Insulin, a hormone generated by the pancreas, operates as a traffic signal, directing glucose cars to your cells.

Insulin connects to receptors on the surface of your cells, acting as a key that unlocks the door. This permits glucose to enter cells and be used for energy production.

Maintaining Balance

This system requires a good blood sugar balance to function properly. Consider rush-hour traffic on the blood sugar freeway. Too much glucose entering the bloodstream at once (e.g., after a sugary meal) might cause traffic congestion. This produces elevated blood sugar levels, also known as hyperglycemia.

The Backup System

But your body has a backup plan. When blood sugar levels rise too high, your pancreas produces more insulin, driving more glucose cars off the highway and into the cells. This helps to lower blood sugar levels back to normal.

The ideal scenario

Ideally, we want traffic to move smoothly on the blood sugar expressway. A well-balanced diet rich in complex carbs (think whole grains, veggies, and fruits) delivers a consistent supply of glucose, avoiding both traffic congestion (high blood sugar) and empty stretches of road (low blood sugar).

Visualizing blood sugar

To help you understand this notion, consider the following analogy:

Think of your blood as a river. The level of the river corresponds to your blood sugar level. A regular flow of water (glucose) keeps the river at an appropriate depth.

Sudden downpours (sugary foods) may cause the river to overflow, resulting in high blood sugar.

Drought conditions (lack of food) may cause the river to dry up, resulting in low blood sugar.

Importance of Balance

Maintaining a good balance is essential for overall health. In the following chapter, we'll go deeper into the realm of carbs, investigating various varieties and their effects on blood sugar. Remember, understanding how your blood sugar system works is the first step toward gaining control!

Now that we have a fundamental grasp of how the blood sugar system works, let us introduce the important characters in this metabolic symphony:

The Star (Glucose): Glucose is the indisputable star of the show, the simple sugar that powers your cells.

Consider it the energy currency widely accepted by your cellular power plants.

Delivery trucks (carbohydrates): Carbohydrates can be thought of as delivery trucks that transfer glucose into the bloodstream. They appear in two major varieties:

Simple carbohydrates: These are similar to fast-food delivery vehicles. They are promptly converted into glucose, resulting in a rapid spike in blood sugar levels. Examples include white bread, sweet beverages, and candies.

Complex Carbohydrates: These are the slow, steady delivery vehicles. They take longer to break down, gradually releasing glucose and improving long-term energy levels. Whole grains, veggies, and fruits are among the examples.

The Traffic Controller (Insulin): This important hormone serves as a traffic controller on the blood sugar highway. It transports glucose from the bloodstream to your cells, maintaining blood sugar levels within a safe range.

The Power Plant (Your Cells): These are the factories that use glucose for energy generation. Consider them independent residences on the blood sugar highway, each requiring a consistent supply of energy to function correctly.

The backup mechanism (the pancreas): This crucial organ serves as a backup mechanism, manufacturing more insulin when blood sugar levels rise too high. It is like having a specialized tow truck on standby to clear traffic congestion on the highway.

Understanding these players and their functions is critical to improving your blood sugar management.

Let's look at some common misunderstandings regarding carbohydrates so you can make better dietary choices that help you achieve your health objectives.

Carbohydrates have received a poor press in recent years, as they are frequently blamed for weight gain and blood sugar issues. However, reality, like most things in life, is complicated. Let's debunk some popular carb myths so you can make more informed choices:

Myth #1: All Carbohydrates Are Bad: This is completely untrue. A balanced diet requires complex carbohydrates, which are found in whole grains, vegetables, and fruits. They supply sustained energy, fiber, and important vitamins and minerals.

Myth #2: Carbohydrates Make You Fat While excessive calorie consumption, regardless of source, can contribute to weight gain, carbs are not the villain. It is the type and quantity of carbohydrates that matter. Refined carbohydrates, such as white bread and sugary drinks, might contribute to weight gain by causing rapid blood sugar rises and subsequent crashes, which enhance hunger desires. Complex carbs, when combined with a balanced diet, can be part of a healthy weight management strategy.

Myth #3: You Should Eliminate Carbs: This can be bad for your health. Carbohydrates are your body's primary source of energy, so restricting yourself can cause weariness, muscular breakdown, and problems concentrating. A balanced approach is essential.

Myth #4: Carbs make you feel sluggish. The contrary is frequently true. Complex carbohydrates provide lasting energy, allowing you to feel energized all day. Simple carbs, on the other hand, can provide a short burst of energy followed by a collapse, resulting in tiredness.

Myth #5: There is no difference between sugar and starch. Both break down into glucose, although at different speeds. Sugar is a simple carbohydrate that is easily absorbed and causes a rapid blood sugar increase. Starch, a complex carbohydrate, takes longer to digest, resulting in a more gradual rise in blood sugar.

Understanding these fallacies and the exact role of carbs is critical for making sound eating decisions. In the following chapter, we will look more closely at the various forms of carbohydrates and how they affect blood sugar. We'll also cover how to identify and select carb sources to help you meet your blood sugar management objectives.

Chapter 3

From Restriction to Empowerment.

Many people who struggle with blood sugar management begin their journey feeling frustrated and limited. Restrictive diets, which promise rapid cures but have an infinite list of rules and foods to avoid, can leave you feeling starved and overwhelmed. What if there was another way? Is there a way to empower yourself with knowledge rather than limitations? This is where carbohydrate counting comes in.

Debunking the Diet Myth

Avoid crash diets and fad trends. These restrictive techniques frequently backfire, resulting in yo-yo dieting, unhealthy connections with food, and, ultimately, a sense of powerlessness. Carbohydrate counting is not a diet; it is a technique. It's about understanding how carbohydrates affect your body and using that information to make informed decisions that help you reach your health goals.

The Power of Knowledge

Imagine strolling into a grocery store armed with the ability to interpret food labels and make informed decisions. Carb counting provides you with this information. You'll learn how to recognize different carbs, calculate their glycemic index (a measure of how quickly they elevate blood sugar), and include them in your meals.

Freedom via Choice

This knowledge turns into freedom. You're no longer confined to a fixed meal plan. Instead, you have the freedom to select from a diverse range of delicious and nutritious foods. Want to have a slice of birthday cake at a party? Carb counting helps you figure it out and make adjustments throughout the day to keep your blood sugar stable.

A personalized approach

Carbohydrate counting is not a one-size-fits-all strategy. Your needs are unique, and your carbohydrate objectives will be determined by a variety of factors, such as your exercise level, weight management goals, and overall health. This book will show you how to set specific carb goals and create a food plan that works for you.

Beyond the Numbers

Carb counting is only one part of the puzzle. This book will also investigate various elements of blood sugar regulation, including the significance of:

Healthy Food Habits: It is critical to maintain a well-balanced diet rich in fruits, vegetables, healthy grains, and lean protein.

Regular Physical Activity: Exercise allows your body to use glucose more efficiently, resulting in better blood sugar control.

Stress Management: Chronic stress can have a harmful impact on blood sugar levels. Meditation and yoga are both useful techniques.

Adequate Sleep: Sleep loss can interfere with hormones that regulate blood sugar. Prioritizing high-quality sleep is key.

Embrace the journey

Carb counting is a voyage of self-discovery. As you explore and discover how different foods affect your blood sugar, you'll develop a better understanding of your body's specific requirements. This knowledge enables you to make informed decisions and take charge of your health, not only in the near term but over your entire life.

In the following chapter, we'll get deeper into the intriguing realm of carbs. We'll look at the many types, their effects on blood sugar, and how to recognize them on food labels. Prepare to learn the secrets of making empowered and informed eating choices!

Chapter 4

Carbohydrates: Friend or Foe?

The Carbohydrate Spectrum

In previous chapters, we discussed the blood sugar roller coaster and the limitations of restrictive diets. Now it's time to go deeper into the world of carbohydrates, separating friends from adversaries and arming you with the information to make sound decisions. Not all carbohydrates are created equal, and recognizing these distinctions is critical to mastering blood sugar management.

The carbohydrate spectrum

Carbohydrates can be generically classified into two types: simple and complicated. Let's look at each type and its effect on blood sugar:

Simple Carbohydrates: These are the "quick energy" carbohydrates, which break down quickly into glucose and cause a sharp rise in blood sugar levels. Consider them as a sugar rush followed by a potential collapse. Here are a few common sources:

Refined sugars: These include table sugar, high-fructose corn syrup, and added sugars found in processed meals, candy, and sugary drinks. They provide little nutritional value and contribute significantly to blood sugar rises.

Starchy Vegetables: While some starchy vegetables, such as maize and peas, include simple carbohydrates, they are frequently accompanied by fiber, which can help slow digestion and regulate blood sugar levels.

Complex carbohydrates are slow and steady energy sources that contain vital elements such as fiber, vitamins, and minerals. They take longer to break down, resulting in a slower rise in blood sugar and sustained energy levels. Here are a few significant sources:

Whole grains: Think brown rice, quinoa, oats, whole-wheat bread, and other unrefined grains. These are high in fiber and essential nutrients, which aid in satiety and blood sugar regulation.

Fruits are nature's candy! Fruits provide natural carbohydrates, fiber, vitamins, and antioxidants. The fiber regulates the absorption of sugar into the bloodstream.

Vegetables: Non-starchy veggies such as leafy greens, broccoli, carrots, and bell peppers are high in vitamins, minerals, and fiber and provide long-lasting energy without causing large blood sugar rises.

The Power of Fiber

Fiber, a complex carbohydrate present in plant-based meals, demands special attention. It works like a magic wand in your digestive system, encouraging a variety of benefits:

Reduces Down Digestion: Fiber promotes satiety and reduces the absorption of glucose into the system, so reducing blood sugar rises.

Promotes stomach health: Fiber feeds the healthy bacteria in your stomach, which improves digestion and overall health.

Fiber keeps you fuller for longer, potentially lowering cravings and assisting with weight management attempts.

Making informed decisions

Understanding the distinction between basic and complex carbohydrates allows you to make more informed eating choices. Here are several important takeaways:

Focus on Complex Carbohydrates: Prioritize complex carbs from whole grains, fruits, and vegetables in your diet. They provide long-lasting energy and necessary nutrients and encourage normal blood sugar levels.

Limit simple carbohydrates: Limit your consumption of refined sugars and processed foods high in simple carbs. These can lead to an increase in blood sugar and leave you feeling exhausted.

Embrace fiber. Look for foods high in fiber, such as whole grains, legumes, and veggies. Fiber is essential for proper digestion, satiety, and blood sugar management.

The Road to Blood Sugar Management

Remember, this is only the beginning of your adventure. In the following chapter, we'll look at practical ways to incorporate these principles into your daily routine. We'll learn how to read food labels effectively, identify healthy substitutions, and develop a meal plan that works for you. By understanding the many types of carbs and their influence on your body, you're well on your way to taking control of your blood sugar and regaining your energy!

Chapter 5

From Knowledge to Action

Practical Strategies for Blood Sugar Management

Welcome back! Now that you have a basic understanding of blood sugar and the significance of carbohydrates, it's time to put that information into practice. This chapter will provide you with practical tactics for navigating grocery store aisles, making smart food choices, and developing a meal plan that meets your blood sugar management objectives.

Decoding food labels like a professional

Food labels can be a wealth of information, but interpreting them can be intimidating. Here's what you should focus on when it comes to carbohydrates:

Total carbohydrates: This value represents the total number of carbs (including simple and complex) in a single dish.

Dietary fiber is your friend! Fiber slows digestion and helps to manage blood sugar. Look for foods with a greater fiber content as compared to total carbs.

Added sugars: Be wary of additional sugars, which can cause blood sugar to rise. Choose foods with little or no added sugar.

Glycemic Index: This index classifies carbs according to their effect on blood sugar. Lower GI foods promote a slower rise in blood sugar, whereas higher GI foods generate faster spikes. While GI is not the only element to consider, it can be a useful tool for making decisions.

Making smart swaps

Small changes in your everyday dietary choices can significantly improve your blood sugar management. Here are several exchanges to consider:

Switch from white bread to whole wheat bread. Whole wheat offers fiber and lasting energy, but white bread can trigger blood sugar surges.

Swap sugary drinks for water or unsweetened tea. Avoid the empty calories and blood sugar spikes that come with sugary drinks.

Swap white rice with brown rice. Brown rice contains more fiber and minerals than white rice.

Snack on fruits and vegetables: These nutrient-dense foods contain both natural sugars and fiber, which promotes balanced blood sugar levels.

Combine carbohydrates, protein, and healthy fats. This combination slows digestion and improves satiety, reducing blood sugar rises. For example, eat an apple with almond butter or scrambled eggs on whole-wheat bread.

Creating a balanced meal plan

Developing a personalized meal plan is critical for long-term success. Here are some suggestions to get you started:

Focus on Portion Control: Even healthy foods might cause blood sugar increases if ingested in excess. Measure glasses and bowls to ensure proper serving sizes.

Plan your meals: Spontaneous decisions frequently result in unhealthy choices. Plan your meals and snacks ahead of time to ensure that you always have healthy options available.

Incorporate Variety: Explore a wide range of complex carbs from several food groups to ensure you're getting all of the nutrients your body requires.

Don't Forget Protein and Healthy Fats: These macronutrients are essential for controlling blood sugar and increasing satiety. Incorporate lean protein sources like chicken, fish, or beans into your meals, as well as healthy fats like avocado, almonds, or olive oil.

Embrace a sustainable approach

Remember that blood sugar management is a marathon, not a sprint. Do not get discouraged by little setbacks. The trick is to focus on progress rather than perfection. Celebrate your accomplishments, big and small, and learn from any mistakes. With constant work and the knowledge you already have, you may develop a long-term strategy for a healthy diet and blood sugar management.

The Road Ahead

The following chapter will go more into the notion of carb counting, which is a useful tool for many people to regulate their blood sugar. We'll look at how to calculate your carbohydrate requirements, track your intake, and use that data to fine-tune your meal plan and improve your health. Stay tuned!

Chapter 6

The Power of Carb Counting

A personalized approach to blood sugar management

In the previous chapter, we looked at practical ways to create a balanced meal plan that promotes appropriate blood sugar levels. This chapter goes into carb counting, a powerful tool for many people concerned about their blood sugar levels. Here, we will reveal the secrets of carb counting, allowing you to tailor your approach to blood sugar management.

Understanding Carbohydrate Counting

Carb counting is tracking how many carbohydrates you ingest throughout the day. This data can then be utilized to make informed dietary choices and forecast how different foods will affect your blood sugar levels. It is not a strict diet, but a flexible approach that allows you to customize your carbohydrate intake based on your specific needs and goals.

Benefits of Carb Counting

While carb counting may appear difficult at first, it has various benefits:

Empowerment and Knowledge: Tracking your carbohydrate intake provides significant insights into how different foods affect your blood sugar. This knowledge enables you to make more educated decisions and take charge of your health.

Improved Blood Sugar Control: Carb counting enables you to modify your carbohydrate consumption to attain and sustain appropriate blood sugar levels. This can dramatically boost your energy and overall well-being.

Flexibility and personalization: Carbohydrate counting is not a one-size-fits-all strategy. You can tailor your carbohydrate consumption to your exercise level, weight management goals, and personal tastes.

Mindful Eating: Tracking carbs promotes mindful eating, which helps you create a better relationship with food.

Getting Started with Carb Counting

Here's a roadmap to help you on your carb-counting journey:

Consult a healthcare professional. Talk to your doctor or registered dietitian about your blood sugar management objectives and the potential benefits of carb counting. They can help you decide whether carb counting is good for you and offer personalized advice.

Set your carbohydrate goals: Your healthcare expert will assist you in setting individualized carbohydrate goals based on your specific demands and health state. These objectives will guide your daily or per-meal carbohydrate intake.

Learn how to read food labels. Learn how to understand the carbohydrate information on food labels. Note total carbohydrates, dietary fiber, and portion sizes.

Invest in tools: There are a variety of tools available to help with carb counting, including phone apps, online resources, and even simple notebooks. Select the technique that best meets your needs and interests.

Carb counting in action

Here's a simple example of how carb counting could function in practice:

Your daily carbohydrate goal is 40 g per meal.

Breakfast: oatmeal (20 g carbs) + berries (5 g carbs) = 25 g total carbs.

This leaves you with 15 grams of carbohydrates for lunch and an additional 15 grams for dinner. As you acquire experience, you'll be able to change portion sizes and meal options to stay within your carb targets.

Remember, carb counting is a journey, not a destination. It requires time, practice, and patience to perfect. Do not get discouraged by little setbacks. The idea is to learn from them and keep pushing for improvement. With constant effort and the instruction provided in this book, you can use carb counting to achieve optimal blood sugar control and uncover a healthier, more energized you!

Based on my professional experience, here are some examples of creating individualized carbohydrate objectives depending on individual needs and health status:

Personalized Carb Goal Examples

Tailoring intake to different needs:

Scenario 1: An active individual with type 2 diabetes.

Individual: John, a 45-year-old male with type 2 diabetes, exercises moderately (30 minutes of brisk walking most days).

Goal: To achieve adequate blood sugar management and maintain a healthy weight.

Carbohydrate Goals (Daily): A daily carbohydrate consumption of approximately 150–200 grams, spread over meals and snacks, may be recommended.

Per meal: This may equate to 45–50 grams of carbs for breakfast, lunch, and dinner, plus 15–20 grams for snacks.

Scenario 2: A pregnant woman has gestational diabetes.

Sarah, a 30-year-old pregnant woman, was diagnosed with gestational diabetes.

Goal: Maintain healthy blood sugar levels for both mother and baby.

Carbohydrate Goals: Daily: To assist embryonic development, a slightly higher daily carbohydrate consumption of 175-200 grams may be recommended.

Per Meal: This might be divided into smaller, more frequent meals and snacks throughout the day, each with 30-45 grams of carbohydrates.

Scenario 3: A person without any blood sugar concerns looking to improve energy levels

Lisa, a 25-year-old woman, frequently experiences afternoon energy drops.

Goal: Increase energy and sustain a healthy lifestyle.

Carbohydrate Goals: Daily: Lisa's doctor may recommend a moderate carbohydrate intake of 130–180 grams per day, depending on her activity level.

Per Meal: She should incorporate complex carbohydrates such as whole grains and veggies throughout the day to provide long-term energy.

Portion sizes would be determined by her unique calorie demands.

Scenario 4: An active teen with no blood sugar issues.

Individual: David, a 16-year-old male athlete participating in everyday sports practice.

Goal: Fuel his body for maximum performance and growth.

Carb Goals: Daily: Given David's high activity level, his doctor may recommend a higher carb consumption of 200–250 grams per day.

Per Meal: This may equate to 50–60 grams of carbs for breakfast and dinner, 30–40 grams for lunch, and carefully placed snacks to provide energy requirements throughout the day.

Scenario 5: A person with prediabetes looking to prevent progression.

Individual: Mary, a 50-year-old woman with prediabetes.

Goal: Improve blood sugar management and avoid the progression of type 2 diabetes.

Mary's doctor may recommend a moderate carbohydrate consumption of 150–180 grams per day, with a focus on complex carbohydrates and portion control.

Per Meal: To avoid blood sugar spikes, she should aim for 40–50 grams of carbs at meals and prioritize healthy snacks containing protein and fiber.

Scenario 6: An elderly person with limited mobility

Individual: Peter is an 80-year-old man with restricted physical activity due to arthritis.

Goal: maintaining appropriate blood sugar levels while controlling calorie consumption.

Carb Goals: For Peter's lower activity level, his doctor may suggest a more restricted carb consumption of 100–130 grams per day.

Per Meal: Smaller, more frequent meals with 25–35 grams of carbohydrates may be useful, with an emphasis on nutrient-dense options to ensure proper vitamin and mineral consumption.

These are only a few examples; actual carbohydrate goals will vary depending on the circumstances. It is critical to speak with a healthcare practitioner to develop a safe and effective carbohydrate intake strategy for your specific needs.

A healthcare professional will create a safe and effective tailored carb intake plan based on your weight, exercise level, blood sugar control goals, and overall health. Other possibilities include:

Scenario 7: Active Individual with Normal Blood Sugar.

James is a 30-year-old man who exercises regularly (imagine daily gym sessions) and has normal blood sugar levels. John's doctor may recommend a daily carbohydrate intake of 180–220 grams, split between meals and snacks. This equates to 45–55 grams per meal and possibly 2-3 snacks containing 15-20 grams of carbs each. The increased intake supports his active lifestyle while maintaining blood sugar management.

Scenario 8: Moderately Active and Prediabetic

Sarah is a 40-year-old lady who works at a desk and enjoys going for walks on occasion. She's been diagnosed with prediabetes. Sarah's doctor may recommend a daily carb goal of 130–150 grams to enhance blood sugar control and prevent the progression of type 2 diabetes. To reduce blood sugar surges, break this down into 30–40 gram servings per meal with smaller, controlled snacks (10–15 grams).

Scenario 9: Less active with type 2 diabetes

David is a 65-year-old guy who enjoys gardening but is limited in mobility because of type 2 diabetes. David's doctor may propose a lower daily carbohydrate consumption of 100–120 grams. To achieve proper blood sugar regulation, divide this into 25–30 gram amounts per meal, with only 5–10 grams of snacking.

Focusing on Specific Goals

Scenario 10: Weight loss

Lisa, a 28-year-old lady, is trying to lose some weight.

Lisa's doctor may propose a daily carb goal of 150–180 grams, besides a reasonable calorie deficit. This might be divided into 40–45-gram portions per meal, with an emphasis on complex carbohydrates and fiber-rich alternatives to enhance satiety and prevent overeating.

Scene 11: Improved Energy Levels

Michael, a 45-year-old man, has afternoon slumps. Michael's doctor might recommend a moderate daily carbohydrate consumption of 160–200 grams, with an emphasis on complex carbs throughout the day. This may equate to 40–50 gram portions per meal, with carefully timed snacks (20–30 grams) combining complex carbs and protein for long-lasting energy.

Navigating the Carb Counting Toolkit

Choosing the Right Tools for You.

Carbohydrate counting does not have to be complicated. There are many tools available to help you track your carbohydrate intake and make smart meal choices. Here's an overview of some popular options to consider:

Phone Applications

Many user-friendly apps include large food databases, barcode scanners for quick product searches, and the ability to track carb intake, blood sugar levels (if applicable), and overall dietary habits. Some even offer tailored carbohydrate target advice and meal-planning tips. Certain apps require a monthly fee. The accuracy of food databases varies, so double-checking product labels is essential. If you prefer a simpler approach, avoid overly complex features. Examples include MyFitnessPal, Lose It!, Carb Manager, and MyPlate by the USDA.

Online Resources

Websites like the American Diabetes Association and the National Institute of Diabetes and Digestive and Kidney Diseases provide free carb counting resources such as food charts, example meal plans, and educational materials. You can also use online carb calculators to estimate your daily carbohydrate requirements.

Navigating and tracking your consumption may require more work than using an app. Personalization is limited when compared to working with a healthcare expert.

Examples include the American Diabetes Association (https://diabetes.org/) and the National Institute of Diabetes and Digestive and Kidney Diseases (https://www.niddk.nih.gov/health-information/diabetes).

Notebooks and spreadsheets

A simple and cost-effective choice that gives you full control over your tracking system. Ideal for people who prefer a pen-and-paper approach or enjoy customizing their tracking system.

Start with what seems most comfortable, and then experiment! You can always take a different approach if necessary. The idea is to discover a technique that will keep you consistent and motivated throughout your carb-counting journey.

Track your intake. Monitor your carbohydrate intake throughout the day. This information will be critical for determining how your body reacts to various foods and fine-tuning your approach.

Chapter 7

Carb counting for each meal

Sample menus and recipes

Now that you have the knowledge and tools for carb counting, it's time to put it into action! This chapter focuses on practical meal-planning tactics, including sample menus and recipes for breakfast, lunch, dinner, and snacks. Remember that these are only examples to get you inspired. Feel free to modify and adjust them according to your own goals, preferences, and dietary requirements.

Strategies for Meal Planning Success

Consider your carbohydrate goals: Refer to the carbohydrate objectives you agreed upon with your healthcare expert. Distribute this consumption strategically over the day's meals and snacks.

Focus on Complex Carbohydrates: Prioritize whole grains, veggies, and fruits for long-lasting energy and healthy blood sugar control.

Pair carbohydrates with protein and healthy fats: This combination enhances satiety and reduces the rise of blood sugar.

Plan: Planning meals and snacks ahead of time reduces the likelihood of making poor decisions at the last minute. Make a grocery list to ensure you have healthy options readily available.

Variety is key: Explore a wide variety of complex carbs from several food groups to ensure you're getting all the nutrients your body requires.

Don't forget to hydrate: Staying hydrated is essential for general health and can keep you feeling fuller for longer.

Sample menus with carb counts (adjust to your particular needs):

Breakfast (30–45 g of carbohydrates):

Option 1: Greek yogurt (15g carbs) topped with berries (10g carbs) and granola (10g carbs).

Option 2: scrambled eggs (2g carbohydrates), whole-wheat bread (20g carbs), and avocado slices (5g carbs).

Lunch (40–50 g carbs):

Option 1: Tuna salad (5g carbohydrates) on a whole-wheat wrap (20g carbs), mixed greens (5g carbs), and a side of cherry tomatoes (5g carbs).

Option 2: lentil soup (25g carbs) served with a side salad (5g carbs) and a whole-wheat bun (15g carbs).

Dinner (45–55 g carbs): Option 1: Salmon (0g carbs) with roasted Brussels sprouts (10g carbs) and quinoa (30g carbs).

Option 2: Stir-fried chicken with brown rice (30g carbohydrates) and mixed vegetables (15g carbs).

Snacks (15–20 g carbohydrates): Option 1: Apple slices (15g carbs) with almond butter (5g carbs).

Option 2: Cottage cheese (5g carbs), chopped vegetables (5g carbs), and a sprinkle of whole-wheat crackers (10g carbs).

Recipe examples:

Whole-wheat pancakes (makes two servings):

Ingredients:

1 cup whole-wheat flour (30 grams of carbohydrates)

1 teaspoon baking powder.

1/4 teaspoon salt.

1 tbsp. Sugar (optional; adjust to liking)

1 egg

1 cup milk (a lactose-free variant is available).

1 tablespoon melted butter or oil.

Instructions:

In a bowl, combine the flour, baking powder, and salt. In a separate bowl, whisk together the egg, milk, and melted butter. Mix the wet and dry ingredients just until mixed (a few lumps are fine). Cook in a lightly oiled skillet over medium heat. Pour the batter in ¼ cup portions into the skillet. Cook for 2-3 minutes on each side, or until golden brown. Serve with your preferred toppings, such as fresh fruit, yogurt, or a sprinkle of maple syrup. Roasted Brussels sprouts with balsamic glaze.

Ingredients:

1 pound of Brussels sprouts, cut and halved

1 tablespoon olive oil.

1/2 teaspoon salt.

1/4 teaspoon black pepper.

2 tablespoons balsamic vinegar.

1 tbsp. Brown sugar (change to preference)

Instructions:

Preheat the oven to 400°F (200°C). On a baking sheet, toss the Brussels sprouts with olive oil, salt, and pepper. Roast for 20–25 minutes, or until tender and gently browned, flipping halfway. In a small saucepan, mix the balsamic vinegar and brown sugar. Bring to a simmer over medium heat, stirring regularly, until somewhat thickened (about 5–7 minutes). Here's your balsamic glaze. Remove the Brussels sprouts from the oven and drizzle with balsamic glaze, stirring to coat evenly. Serve immediately. (Estimated carbohydrates per serving: 10 g)

Breakfast (30–45 g of carbohydrates):

Power Breakfast Bowl (35 grams of carbohydrates):

Mix 1/2 cup cooked oatmeal (30g carbs) with a scoop of protein powder (5g carbs), a handful of berries (5g carbs), and a dab of nut butter (5g carbs) for a protein-packed and tasty start to the day.

Savory Frittata (30 grams of carbohydrates):

Saute chopped veggies such as onions, peppers, and spinach (5 grams of carbohydrates).

Whisk together the eggs (2g carbohydrates), milk (lactose-free option available), and cheese (5g carbs).

Pour the egg mixture over the vegetables in a skillet and heat until done.

This protein-rich, vegetable-packed alternative is ideal for breakfast or a light lunch.

Lunch (40–50 g carbs):

Mediterranean Chickpea Salad Sandwich (40 grams of carbohydrates):

Chickpeas (25g carbs) and chopped veggies such as tomatoes, cucumbers, and red onion (5g carbs) are mixed with a tasty vinaigrette dressing (5g carbs) and served on whole-wheat pita bread (10g carbs). This vegetarian option is packed with protein and fiber.

Black Bean Burgers (35g carbs):

Combine cooked black beans (20g carbs) with chopped onion, bell pepper (5g carbs), and spices.

Form into patties and cook on the grill or in a pan.

Serve on whole-wheat buns (10 grams of carbohydrates each) with lettuce, tomato, and a light spray of your favorite sauce. This tasty plant-based choice is high in protein and fiber.

Dinner (45–55 g carbohydrates):

Salmon with Lemon Dill Sauce and Roasted Asparagus (40 grams of carbohydrates):

Bake fish (0g carbohydrates), drizzled with olive oil and lemon juice. In a separate skillet, roast the asparagus (5 grams of carbohydrates) with salt and pepper. For a light and tasty supper, top the salmon with a simple sauce comprising fresh dill, lemon juice, and a small amount of low-fat yogurt (5 grams of carbohydrates).

Turkey Chili with Brown Rice (50g carbs): sauté ground turkey with chopped vegetables such as onions, peppers, and corn (10g carbs). Combine canned chopped tomatoes, kidney beans (15 grams of carbohydrates), chili powder, and other spices. Simmer for a minimum of 30 minutes. Serve overcooked brown rice (30 grams of carbohydrates) for a substantial and warm meal.

Snacks with 15-20 grams of carbohydrates include edamame with chili flakes (15 grams of carbs).

A simple yet tasty snack alternative. Edamame pods include plant-based protein and fiber.

To add some spice, sprinkle with a pinch of chili flakes.

Greek Yogurt Parfait (18 g carbohydrates):

For a protein-packed and tasty snack: combine 1/2 cup plain Greek yogurt (10g carbs) with a handful of mixed berries (5g carbs) and a sprinkling of chopped nuts (3g carbs).

These are only the beginning points. The second edition of this book delves into over 100 delicious, carb-conscious recipes that are tailored to your dietary goals and preferences.

Remember that these are just estimates; the real carb amount will vary depending on the ingredients, brand, and serving size. Always check food labels for the correct carb levels. Don't be scared to get creative in the kitchen and make your own nutritious and delicious carb-conscious foods. The idea is to prioritize complex carbohydrates, combine them with protein and healthy fats, and be cautious of portion amounts. With creativity and these guiding principles, you can embark on a delicious journey to good blood sugar management.

Chapter 8

Create Your Personalized Carb Budget for Blood Sugar Success.

Carb counting is an effective strategy for managing blood sugar, but it must be tailored to the individual. A one-size-fits-all solution does not exist. This chapter will walk you through the process of building a personalized carb budget based on your activity level, health goals, and particular needs.

Understand Your Baseline

Before creating a carb budget, you must first understand your current carb intake. There are two basic approaches for accomplishing this.

Food journaling: For one week, precisely document everything you eat and drink, including the approximate carbohydrate amount. You can use a variety of apps and internet tools to calculate this.

Analyzing your meal log will reveal your daily carbohydrate intake.

Continuous Glucose Monitoring: If you have access to a CGM, you can get real-time input on how different diets and activities affect your blood sugar. This knowledge can be quite useful in understanding how your body responds to carbs.

Consider your activity level

Your exercise level has a big impact on your carbohydrate requirements. Here's the breakdown:

Sedentary Lifestyle: People who do less physical exercise need fewer carbs (about 100–150 grams per day).

Moderately Active: People who engage in frequent moderate-intensity exercise (such as brisk walking or swimming) may require a modest carb budget (150–200 grams per day).

Highly Active: Those who engage in strenuous exercise or sports training frequently demand a higher carbohydrate budget (up to 250 grams or more per day) to fuel their efforts and aid recuperation.

Examples on customized carb budget

Assume you now consume an average of 220 grams of carbohydrates per day and have a moderately active lifestyle that includes daily walks and the occasional gym session.

Based on this information, make a baseline adjustment. Given your current intake (220 grams) and somewhat active lifestyle, a daily reduction of 20–30 grams appears feasible. This amounts to a daily target carbohydrate intake of approximately 190–200 grams.

Assume your primary goal is to enhance blood glucose management. In this situation, a target of 190 grams per day is appropriate for your activity level and allows for progressive adjustment based on your blood sugar reaction.

Here's your customized carb budget based on the example.

Target carb intake: 190 grams per day.

Implementing Your Carbohydrate Budget: Now comes the exciting part: putting your carb budget into action! Here's how to divide your daily carb intake across meals and snacks:

Breakfast (30–40 grams): Choose a balanced breakfast with a moderate carbohydrate supply, such as whole-wheat toast with eggs and veggies or Greek yogurt with berries and a sprinkling of granola.

Lunch (50–60 grams): Try a salad with grilled chicken or fish, brown rice with lean protein and roasted vegetables, or a whole-wheat wrap with hummus and veggies.

Dinner (60 to 70 grams): Prepare a supper dish with grilled salmon, chicken breast, or vegetarian chili, roasted veggies, and a small serving of quinoa or brown rice.

Snacks (2-3 snacks, 10-20 g each): Choose nutritious snacks such as apple slices with almond butter, a handful of mixed nuts with dried cranberries, or vegetable sticks with Greek yogurt dip.

Remember, this is only a sample breakdown. You can change the portion sizes and carbohydrate sources to suit your preferences and needs.

Tracking Your Progress

Monitoring your progress is essential for fine-tuning your carb budget. Here are a few methods:

Food journaling: Keeping a detailed meal record allows you to monitor your daily carb intake and find potential areas for improvement.

Carb Counting Applications: Several phone apps can make carb tracking easier by giving nutritional information for a variety of foods.

Blood Sugar Monitoring: If you have diabetes or prediabetes, checking your blood sugar levels before and after meals can indicate how your body reacts to different carbohydrate intakes.

Tuning Your Carb Budget

Consider the following when implementing your carb budget:

Blood Sugar Response: If your blood sugar levels are regularly high, consider reducing your daily carb intake. In contrast, if you feel regular weariness or difficulties managing hunger, a small increase may be required.

Activity Level: If your activity level drastically increases, you may need to raise your carb budget to ensure that you have enough fuel for your workouts.

Individual Needs: Everyone's body reacts differently to carbs. Be patient, experiment, and adjust your carbohydrate budget based on your specific needs and how you feel.

Creating your carbohydrate budget is a positive step toward regulating your blood sugar and achieving your health goals. Remember that consistency is crucial. Track your progress, alter your carbohydrate budget as needed, and celebrate your accomplishments along the way. With devotion and these useful tools, you may enter a world of healthy living and enhanced blood sugar control.

Chapter 9

The Art of Portion Control

Mastering Bite Without Feeling Deprived

Portion control is essential for healthy eating, and it is especially important for individuals who are diabetic. This chapter provides you with useful ways to control portion sizes without feeling confined or deprived.

The Power of Portion Control

Beyond blood sugar management, portion control provides a plethora of benefits.

Weight Management: Consuming enough calories is critical for maintaining a healthy weight. Portion control allows you to avoid exceeding your daily calorie requirements.

Improved Satiety: Eating nutrient-dense foods and adhering to recommended portion sizes can increase feelings of fullness and satisfaction, lowering cravings and preventing overeating.

Developing a mindful approach to portion control promotes a healthy connection with food by instilling intuitive eating habits and a sense of control.

Understanding Portion Sizes Without Deprivation

The key to successful portion management is not feeling like you're always on a rigid diet. Here are some practical strategies for accomplishing this:

Downsize Your Dishes: Using smaller plates and bowls offers a sense of abundance, even when serving fewer servings. A smaller dish brimming with nutritious food can be more psychologically fulfilling than a large platter with a modest serving.

Embrace Your Hands: Use your hand as a guide for portion size. A cupped hand roughly equals one meal of cooked grains or pasta, whereas your palm represents one portion of protein. This is a convenient and portable method for estimating portions on the move.

Check the food labels: Pay special attention to the portion sizes specified on food labels. This is an excellent starting point for portion management, particularly for prepackaged foods.

Measure Until You Memorize: Begin by familiarizing yourself with acceptable portion sizes for various food groups using measuring cups and spoons. Over time, you'll develop an instinctive sense of portion management and won't require the measurement instruments as often.

Focus on Nutrient Density: Eat complete, unprocessed meals that are naturally satisfying. These foods offer more volume and enjoyment for fewer calories. Nutrient-dense foods such as vegetables, fruits, and whole grains keep you satiated for longer, lowering the desire to overeat.

Slow down and appreciate your food. Allow your body to receive fullness cues. Mindful eating activities help you become more aware of your body's cues and avoid overconsumption.

Plan Your Meals: Preparing meals and snacks ahead of time reduces impulsive decisions and allows you to regulate portion size. When you have healthy options easily available, you're less likely to reach for bad snacks when hunger strikes.

Mindful eating practices include paying attention to hunger and fullness indicators. Stop eating when you are comfortably full, not stuffed. Mindful eating allows you to appreciate your food while avoiding excessive calorie intake.

Allow yourself to indulge in moderation. Deprivation can trigger cravings and overeating. Concentrate on conscious enjoyment. To build a sustainable and satisfying eating routine, have a lesser piece of your favorite indulgence occasionally rather than eliminating it.

Make Healthy Swaps: When cravings strike, consider healthier options. Replace sugary drinks with sparkling water and fruit slices, or eat a little square of dark chocolate instead of a huge candy bar.

Remember that portion control is a journey, not a destination. Be patient with yourself and applaud your accomplishments. There will be days when you overeat, which is fine. The idea is to learn from these experiences and recommit to mindful eating habits.

Mastering portion control and developing mindful eating habits are critical components of maintaining good blood sugar levels and general well-being. Using the principles outlined in this chapter, you can develop a balanced and sustainable approach to food, allowing you to take control of your health. Remember, consistency and a personalized strategy are essential for success on your path to mindful eating and maximum health.

Chapter 10

Fiber Factor

Friend of Blood Sugar Control

Dietary fiber, sometimes known as the "bulky" element of plant-based foods, is essential for digestion, gut health, and, most crucially, blood sugar management. This chapter looks into the science of how fiber affects blood sugar levels and shows how to incorporate it into your carb calculations for a more nuanced result.

Understanding Fiber and Blood Sugar

Unlike other carbs, the human body cannot fully digest and absorb fiber. Here's how it affects blood glucose:

Fiber slows digestion by adding weight to meals, which delays stomach emptying and glucose (blood sugar) absorption into the bloodstream. This results in a slower rise in blood sugar levels, which promotes improved overall blood sugar control.

Feeding stomach bacteria: Fiber serves as a prebiotic, supporting the beneficial bacteria in your stomach. These helpful bacteria convert fiber into short-chain fatty acids (SCFAs), which may improve insulin sensitivity and contribute to healthy blood sugar regulation.

Types of Fiber and Their Impact on Blood Sugar

There are two major forms of fiber, each with its unique impact on blood sugar.

Soluble fiber dissolves in water and forms a gel-like material in the digestive tract. Soluble fiber is very beneficial in delaying digestion and lowering blood sugar levels. Examples include oat beta-glucan, psyllium husk, and apple pectin.

Insoluble fiber does not dissolve in water but adds weight to feces, improving regularity. While it does not directly affect blood sugar absorption, it can increase feelings of satiety, lowering overall calorie intake and indirectly benefiting blood sugar management. Examples include cellulose from vegetables and bran.

Factoring Fiber into Carb Counting

Because fiber has little effect on blood sugar, some carb-counting methods classify it as "net carbs." Here's how to calculate net carbohydrates:

Net carbs are total carbs minus dietary fiber.

For example, if a portion of brown rice contains 30 grams of total carbohydrates and 2 grams of dietary fiber, the net carbs are 28 grams (30 grams minus 2 grams). This enables you to concentrate on the carbohydrates that directly affect your blood sugar levels.

Important considerations

Check Food Labels: Nowadays, most food labels list both total carbs and dietary fiber amounts. Use this information to calculate the net carbohydrates in packaged goods.

Consult a health professional. While the net carb approach might be beneficial, consult with your doctor or registered dietitian to ensure that it meets your specific needs and health goals.

Focus on Whole Foods: Choose whole, unprocessed foods that are naturally high in fiber. These foods often have a lower glycemic index (GI), which means they induce a slower rise in blood sugar than refined carbohydrates.

Fiber is an effective ally in your blood sugar management quest. Understanding its benefits and properly combining them into your carb-counting technique can help you construct a long-term and effective plan for optimal health. Remember, consistency and a personalized approach are essential. Consult your healthcare expert for personalized advice on incorporating fiber and net carbs into your carb-counting plan.

With the knowledge gained in this chapter, you'll be able to confidently navigate the realm of carb counting. Remember, this is a journey, and there will be changes along the way. Embrace the process, appreciate your achievements, and empower yourself to take control of your health with mindful eating habits.

Chapter 11

The Exercise Equation

Balancing blood sugar and physical activity

Physical activity is an essential component of a healthy lifestyle, and for those managing blood sugar levels, it becomes an even more effective tool. This chapter digs into the science of how exercise affects blood sugar and discusses tactics for modifying carb intake to improve workouts and blood sugar control.

Exercise and Blood Sugar.

Exercise has a variety of benefits for blood sugar management, including:

Increased glucose uptake: During physical exertion, your muscles use glucose (blood sugar) as energy. This increased demand might cause a drop in blood sugar levels, especially after exercise.

Improved Insulin Sensitivity: Regular exercise increases your body's sensitivity to insulin, a hormone that transports glucose from the bloodstream to the cells. This higher insulin sensitivity enables your body to use glucose more efficiently, resulting in better blood sugar control.

Enhanced Glycemic Control: Exercise can help your body balance blood sugar levels more effectively. This results in more consistent blood sugar levels throughout the day, even during and after exercise.

Timing and type of pre-exercise meal or snack can affect workout performance and blood sugar regulation. Here are some important considerations to consider:

Timing: Aim to have a snack or meal 30–60 minutes before your workout. This gives your body enough time to digest and absorb nutrients, allowing you to workout with maximum vitality.

Carbohydrate content: The amount of carbohydrates required before exercise is determined by several factors, including the intensity and duration of your workout, your blood sugar objectives, and how long it has been since your previous meal. Typically, a moderate-intensity activity lasting less than an hour may necessitate a modest snack containing 15-20 grams of carbohydrates. For longer or more difficult workouts, a bigger snack or supper containing 30-45 grams of carbohydrates may be recommended.

Glycemic Index (GI): Choose low-GI carbs for your pre-workout meal or snack. Low-GI alternatives gently release glucose into the bloodstream, delivering sustained energy during your workout while reducing blood sugar spikes. Whole grains, low-GI fruits such as berries, and vegetables are among the examples.

Protein and Healthy Fats: Including a reasonable quantity of protein and healthy fats in your pre-workout meal or snack will help boost long-term energy and satiety. Nuts, nut butter, fruit-flavored yogurt, and a hard-boiled egg with whole-wheat bread are some examples.

Blood sugar monitoring is critical for diabetics and anyone who experiences large variations after exercise. Here's how it helps:.

Identify pre-exercise needs: Checking your blood sugar before exercising can help you identify whether you require a pre-workout snack to avoid hypoglycemia (low blood sugar) during your workout.

Track your blood sugar reaction after exercise to see how your body reacts to different types and amounts of pre-workout meals or snacks. This information can help you fine-tune your strategy for maximum control.

Adjusting Carbohydrate Intake Based on Exercise

The intensity and duration of your exercise program will affect your carbohydrate requirements. This is a general guide:

Low-Intensity Exercise: Activities such as mild strolling or moderate yoga may not require considerable carbohydrate changes. However, it is still essential to monitor your blood sugar.

Moderate-Intensity Exercise: For workouts that last less than an hour, a short pre-workout snack containing 15-20 grams of carbs may be required. A light snack high in protein and carbohydrates can aid recuperation after exercise.

High-Intensity or Long-Duration Exercise: For strenuous workouts lasting more than an hour, a bigger pre-workout breakfast of 30-45 grams of carbs may be required. A balanced breakfast containing carbohydrates, protein, and healthy fats is recommended after an exercise to help with muscle repair and glycogen replenishment.

Remember that these are general principles. Your appropriate carbohydrate intake will be determined by your particular demands and activity schedule.

Consulting with a qualified dietitian or healthcare expert can assist you in developing a specific carbohydrate intake plan based on your activity patterns and blood sugar targets.

Additional considerations

Medication adjustments: If you take diabetes medications, your doctor may need to change your dosage based on your exercise schedule to prevent hypoglycemia.

Hydration: Staying hydrated is essential for peak performance and blood sugar regulation while exercising. Drink plenty of water before, during, and following your workout.

Listen to your body: Pay attention to how you feel during and after exercising. If you get hypoglycemia symptoms such as dizziness, shakiness, or confusion while working out, stop and ingest a quick-acting carbohydrate such as juice or glucose tablets.

There is no one-size-fits-all solution to exercise and carbohydrate intake. Experiment with various pre-workout meals, snacks, and post-workout recovery options while tracking your blood sugar levels. This tailored approach will assist you in determining what works best for your physique and exercise routine.

The Synergy of Exercise and Carb Management

Understanding how exercise affects blood sugar and deliberately modifying your carbohydrate intake can result in a powerful synergy. This combination improves your exercise, promotes improved blood sugar control, and gives you the ability to maintain your health properly.

This chapter has taught you how to navigate the relationship between exercise and carbohydrate management. Remember that consistency is crucial. As you incorporate physical exercise into your routine and improve your carbohydrate intake plan, you'll feel the countless benefits of this powerful combination.

Exercise and carbohydrate management are effective methods for improving your health and well-being. By may control your blood sugar, increase your energy levels, and reach your fitness goals by engaging in physical activity and eating carbohydrates with caution. Remember, this is a journey, and there will be changes along the way. Celebrate your accomplishments, embrace the learning process, and empower yourself to live a bright and healthy lifestyle.

Chapter 12

Meds and Carbs

Navigating Interactions for Best Blood Sugar Control

Navigating the interplay between drugs and carbs becomes a key element of successful blood sugar control for those who are using medication. This chapter investigates possible interactions between common blood sugar drugs and carbs, as well as methods for adjusting your carb-counting approach for the best outcomes.

Medicine Interactions

Blood sugar control drugs operate in different ways. Here's a breakdown of several common drugs and their possible interactions with carbohydrates:

Metformin: This medicine improves insulin sensitivity and lowers glucose synthesis in the liver. Metformin does not cause hypoglycemia (low blood sugar) on its own; however, ingesting too few carbohydrates or exercising excessively without modifying your carb intake can result in hypoglycemia when on metformin.

Sulfonylureas: These drugs cause the pancreas to secrete more insulin. Consuming too many carbohydrates or skipping meals can cause hypoglycemia when using sulfonylureas. Conversely, eating too few carbohydrates can make them useless.

DPP-4 Inhibitors (Gliptins): These drugs act through incretin, which are natural gut chemicals that promote insulin release after a meal while decreasing glucagon synthesis. DPP-4 inhibitors have a low risk of hypoglycemia, but they may promote weight gain if not accompanied by a good diet and exercise.

SGLT2 Inhibitors: These drugs prevent the kidneys from reabsorbing glucose, allowing excess glucose to be discharged into the urine. SGLT2 inhibitors can result in urinary tract infections and dehydration. Staying hydrated is essential when using these drugs.

Importance of Medication Disclosure

When discussing carb counting with your healthcare practitioner, make sure to reveal all the drugs you're taking, including those that aren't especially for blood sugar control. This detailed information enables your doctor or registered dietitian to adjust your carb-counting plan to minimize potential interactions with drugs.

Strategies for Adjusting Carb Counting with Medications

Here are some techniques to consider when tailoring your carb-counting strategy to your medications:

Consistent carbohydrate consumption: Aims for steady carbohydrate consumption throughout the day. This allows your body to anticipate insulin release, reducing blood sugar spikes and drops. It is critical to distribute carbohydrates equally throughout your meals and snacks.

Focus on including fiber-rich carbs in your diet. Fiber delays digestion and carbohydrate absorption, resulting in a more gradual rise in blood glucose.

Glycemic Index (GI) matters: Choose low-GI carbs wherever possible. Low-GI alternatives gradually release glucose into the system, reducing blood sugar spikes and improving overall glycemic control.

Monitor Blood Sugar: Regular blood sugar monitoring is especially crucial while starting a new medication or changing your carbohydrate intake. Monitoring allows you to spot potential interactions and alter your carb-counting method.

Working With Your Healthcare Team

Effective blood sugar management necessitates coordination with your healthcare team. Here's how they can help you:

Personal Carb Counting Plan: Your doctor or certified dietitian can assist you in developing a personalized carb-counting strategy based on your medication regimen, individual needs, and lifestyle considerations.

Medication Adjustments: If your blood sugar management does not improve after changes to your carb-counting method, your doctor may need to adjust your medication dosage or type.

Ongoing Support: Your healthcare team can help you negotiate the interactions between medications, carb intake, and blood sugar control.

Additional considerations include **sick days,** which might impact blood sugar control. Inform your doctor of any changes in your health, and adjust your carbohydrate consumption and medication regimen as necessary.

Travel and Time Changes: Traveling can break your normal schedule. Plan your meals and snacks ahead of time, and consider changing your carbohydrate consumption or prescription regimen to account for time zone variations.

Stress Management: Chronic stress can raise blood sugar levels. To reduce the influence of stress on blood sugar regulation, use practices such as yoga, meditation, or deep breathing.

Managing blood sugar levels with drugs complicates your carb-counting journey. However, it does not have to be overpowering. Understanding potential interactions, collaborating with your healthcare team, and changing your carb-counting technique will help you negotiate this element of blood sugar control successfully. Remember that consistency, open communication with your doctor, and a dedication to healthy behaviors are essential for maintaining optimal blood sugar management and a fulfilling life.

Chapter 13

Dining Out Without Disaster

Mastering the Menu for Blood Sugar Success.

Navigating restaurant menus can feel like entering unfamiliar territory for individuals managing their blood sugar levels. However, with the appropriate methods, you may turn dining out from a possible disaster into a pleasant and blood sugar-friendly experience. This chapter provides you with the necessary skills to make educated decisions and enjoy great meals without jeopardizing your health goals.

A Plan for Success

Preparation is essential for a seamless and pleasurable dining experience. Here are some preemptive strategies:

Research the menu: Nowadays, many restaurants offer their menus online. Browse the menu ahead of time to find healthy selections that meet your carb-counting objectives and tastes.

Consider Portion Sizes: Restaurant meals are notoriously enormous. Be mindful of portion sizes and consider splitting a dish or bringing half of your meal home for later.

Pack smart snacks: If you are concerned about the restaurant's healthy alternatives, bring a low-carb, high-protein snack, such as nuts or sugar-free yogurt, to keep you content until you can make a good decision.

Menu Navigation Strategy

Once you're at the restaurant, these strategies will lead you to blood sugar-friendly options:

Focus on Protein: Prioritize lean protein sources such as grilled chicken, fish, and tofu. Protein keeps you satisfied for longer and can help prevent blood sugar increases after eating carbohydrates.

Embrace Vegetables: Vegetables are low in carbs and high in key nutrients. To cut out on additional fats and sugars, choose steamed, grilled, or roasted vegetables.

Remember the sauces and dressings? Restaurant sauces and dressings are frequently filled with hidden sugars and bad fats. Request dressings and sauces on the side, or ask for a vinaigrette.

Go bun-less: If your burger or sandwich comes with a bun, consider eating the patties or filling on their own, or request a lettuce wrap instead of a bun.

Beware of hidden sugars: Be aware of ostensibly nutritious recipes that may include hidden sweets. Salads containing candied nuts or dried fruit, as well as "healthy" sauces like teriyaki or barbecue, can contain surprising amounts of sugar. If you're unsure, ask your server about the ingredients.

Do not be afraid to ask questions. Don't be afraid to ask questions about ingredients and cooking procedures. Most eateries are willing to accommodate dietary requirements. Inquire about substitutes or changes to make a dish healthy.

Healthy Appetizer and Entrée Examples

Here are some blood sugar-friendly appetizer and entrée options to consider:

Appetizers: edamame, grilled shrimp cocktail, steaming veggie dumplings, or a small serving of guacamole on whole-wheat pita.

Entrees include grilled salmon with roasted vegetables, chicken stir-fry with brown rice (request light sauce), a veggie burger on a whole-wheat bun with a side salad (dressing on the side), steak with a baked sweet potato (reserve a small portion of the sweet potato), and tofu scramble with sautéed vegetables.

Dessert Considerations

While having dessert occasionally is completely appropriate, here are some healthier options to consider.

Fruit plate: A small fruit plate sprinkled with almonds or a dollop of plain yogurt will satisfy your sweet desire without causing a big blood sugar surge.

Unsweetened tea or coffee with milk or cream is a low-carb, satisfying way to finish your meal.

Portion Control: If you choose a higher-carb dessert, share it with a friend or family member, or take half of it home for later.

Dining out does not need to be a blood sugar nightmare. You may have tasty and enjoyable restaurant meals without jeopardizing your health objectives by planning ahead of time, using these menu navigation skills, and making informed decisions.

Additional Tips

Bring your low-carb condiments: If you have trouble finding healthy dressing options, bring a tiny packet of your favorite low-carb salad dressing.

Hydration is key: Staying hydrated throughout your meal aids digestion and might lead to feelings of fullness. Choose water or unsweetened iced tea over sugary drinks.

Mindful Eating: Pay attention to hunger and fullness signs. Eat deliberately and relish your meals, ending when you're comfortably full, not stuffed.

Dining out may be a great social event. By implementing these tactics and making informed decisions, you can turn restaurant meals into opportunities to try new flavors, spend time with loved ones, and confidently navigate your blood sugar management journey. Remember, consistency.

Chapter 14

Beyond the Numbers

A comprehensive approach to blood sugar management Blood sugar management is frequently reduced to three numbers: blood sugar levels, carbohydrate intake, and prescription dosages. While these data are significant, a truly holistic approach to blood sugar control extends beyond the measures. This chapter investigates the role of sleep, stress management, and self-care in achieving good blood sugar health and general well-being.

Sleep and Blood Sugar

Sleep regulates hormones that affect blood sugar regulation. Here's how.

Insulin sensitivity: Chronic sleep deprivation can reduce insulin sensitivity, making it difficult for your body to use insulin properly and resulting in high blood sugar levels.

Stress Hormones: A lack of sleep impairs the production of stress hormones such as cortisol. Elevated cortisol levels can stimulate glucagon release, a hormone that raises blood sugar levels.

Sleep deprivation can affect appetite-regulating hormones such as leptin (which promotes satiety) and ghrelin (which raises hunger). This might cause increased desires and overeating, compromising blood sugar management.

The Sleep You Need

The National Sleep Foundation suggests that individuals receive 7-9 hours of good sleep per night. Prioritizing proper sleep hygiene activities can dramatically improve your sleep quality.

Establish a regular sleep schedule. Go to bed and get up at consistent times, even on weekends. This helps to regulate your body's normal sleep-wake cycle.

Create a relaxing bedtime routine: Create a peaceful bedtime ritual, such as having a warm bath, reading a book, or practicing relaxation techniques. Avoid stimulating activities, such as screen time, before bedtime.

Optimize Your Sleep Environment: To promote restful sleep, keep your bedroom dark, quiet, cool, and clear of clutter.

Limit Caffeine and Alcohol Consumption: Avoid drinking too much caffeine, especially in the afternoon and evening, as it might interfere with sleep. Limit your alcohol consumption because it can interfere with your sleep quality.

Regular physical activity can help enhance sleep quality. However, avoid intense exercise too close to bedtime because it can be arousing.

Chronic stress can negatively impact blood sugar levels. Here's why.

Stress Hormone Release: In stressful situations, your body produces cortisol and adrenaline. These hormones can raise blood sugar levels, providing readily available energy for the "fight or flight" response.

Blood Sugar Regulation: Chronic stress can affect the body's capacity to manage blood sugar properly. Over time, this can cause insulin resistance and high blood sugar levels.

Effective stress management is essential for maintaining appropriate blood sugar levels.

Identify your stressors. The first step is to identify the situations or things that cause stress in your life. Keeping a stress diary can help with this process.

Deep breathing, meditation, yoga, and progressive muscle relaxation are among the relaxation practices that can help you handle stress at the moment.

Mindfulness techniques: Mindfulness techniques such as mindful meditation can help you become more aware of your thoughts and feelings, allowing you to deal with stress more constructively.

Seek Support: Do not be afraid to seek help from friends, family, a therapist, or a support group. Talking about your stress might be an effective way to handle it.

Prioritize a healthy lifestyle: that includes frequent exercise, a balanced diet, and adequate sleep. These routines improve overall well-being and resilience to stress.

Self-care is crucial for managing blood sugar and maintaining overall health. Here's how.

Listen to your body: Pay heed to your body's hunger and fullness signals. Eat when you're hungry and quit when you're full. Do not deprive yourself, but be cautious of your portion amounts and dietary choices.

Stay hydrated: Drinking plenty of water throughout the day keeps you hydrated, promotes a sense of fullness, and can help with blood sugar regulation.

Move your body: Regular physical activity is an essential component of blood sugar regulation. Find activities you enjoy and incorporate them into your daily routine.

Enjoy Life: Schedule time for things you find enjoyable and soothing. Laughter, quality time with loved ones, and hobbies can all help to reduce stress and improve general well-being.

Celebrate your successes: Recognize and appreciate your accomplishments, no matter how minor. A positive mindset is vital for staying motivated on your blood sugar management path.

Chapter 15

You Got This!

Embracing Motivation and Celebrating Achievements in Your Blood Sugar Management Journey

Congratulations! By reaching this chapter, you've begun a strong journey to regain control of your blood sugar and improve your health. This chapter discusses ways to stay motivated, recognize your accomplishments, and cultivate a positive and empowered mentality throughout your blood sugar management journey.

Maintaining motivation: Keep the Flame Alive

Motivation is the fuel that propels you along your health path. Here are some suggestions to keep your motivational fire blazing brightly:

Set SMART goals. Set specific, measurable, achievable, relevant, and time-bound goals. Setting small, attainable goals allows you to celebrate your accomplishments frequently and stay motivated. For example, instead of setting a general goal of "eating healthier," try to include one more serving of veggies in your regular meals for one week.

Find your "why": Connect with your underlying purpose for controlling your blood sugar. Is it to boost your energy, avoid future health issues, or simply feel better overall? When confronted with a task, having a clear "why" can be an effective motivator.

Embrace progress, not perfection. There will be bumps in the road. Do not allow failures to hinder your development. Focus on appreciating little victories and learning from mistakes. Remember, consistency is more important than perfection.

Find a support system: Surround yourself with positive, supporting individuals. Connect with friends, family, or online communities that understand your situation and can provide encouragement.

Reward yourself: Celebrate your accomplishments with nutritious rewards. After hitting a milestone, treat yourself to a relaxing massage or get new training attire to help you achieve your fitness goals. These rewards encourage positive conduct and keep you engaged.

Celebrating Successes: Large or Small, They All Matter.

Celebrating your accomplishments, no matter how minor, is essential for staying motivated and developing a positive self-image. Here's how to transform your victories into stepping stones:

Acknowledge your achievements: Take time to recognize and appreciate your progress. Did you follow your healthy eating plan for a week? Did you add a new sort of exercise to your routine? Celebrate these victories!

Track your progress: Keeping a notebook or using a progress tracker app allows you to visualize your path and celebrate both major and minor milestones. Seeing tangible evidence of your hard work can be quite motivating.

Share Your Victories: Share your accomplishments with supportive friends, family, or online communities. Sharing your triumphs might help you gain confidence and inspire others.

Focus on Your Feelings: Beyond the numbers, enjoy how you feel as you move forward on your path. Have you got extra energy? Do you sleep better? Concentrate on the positive changes in your well-being.

Treat yourself in a healthy way. Reward yourself with healthy goodies as you meet milestones. Enjoy a low-sugar smoothie after meeting a workout goal, or reward yourself with a relaxing spa day following weeks of continuous good eating.

The Power of Positivity: cultivating a growth mindset.

Having a positive and growth-oriented mindset is critical for long-term success. Here's how you can build this empowering mindset:

Embrace challenges. View challenges as opportunities for learning and development. Setbacks are not failures, but stepping stones towards advancement.

Self-compassion is key. Be gentle with yourself. Forgive yourself for occasional mistakes and refocus on your goals. Self-compassion improves emotional well-being and increases motivation.

Focus on Progress: Rather than concentrating on past mistakes, consider the progress you're making. Track your progress and celebrate your accomplishments.

Visualization is powerful. Spend time imagining yourself accomplishing your blood sugar management objectives. Mentally rehearse healthy activities and imagine yourself at your finest. Visualization might help you gain drive and concentrate.

Believe in yourself: Develop a strong belief in your capacity to control your blood sugar and meet your health objectives. Your self-belief is a tremendous force that can move you forward in your life.

You are in charge of your blood sugar management journey. You can achieve optimal health and well-being by using the principles provided in this book, focusing on a holistic approach, and cultivating a positive and empowered mindset. Remember to enjoy your accomplishments, learn from disappointments, and believe in your potential to thrive. You have got this!

Bonus Chapter

Carb Counting Champions

Real People, Real Results

Real-life tales can be more motivating than numbers on a page. This additional chapter showcases the inspiring stories of people who have successfully used carb counting to control their blood sugar and improve their health.

Meet Sarah. From Frustration to Freedom.

Sarah, a busy marketing professional, was diagnosed with type 2 diabetes a few years ago. After becoming overwhelmed and dissatisfied with restrictive diets, she discovered carb counting. "It was a revelation," she explains. "I finally understood how food impacted my blood sugar, and I could make informed choices without feeling deprived." Sarah learned how to navigate restaurant menus, manage social gatherings, and enjoy a wide range of foods by measuring carbohydrates. "It's not about deprivation," she says, "but about empowerment. I control my blood sugar, not the other way around."

Key takeaways from Sarah's story:

Carb counting enables you to make more educated dietary decisions.

It enables flexibility and the enjoyment of a wide range of foods.

Blood sugar management focuses on control rather than restriction.

Meet David: rekindling his passion for life

David, an active grandfather, observed a drop in his energy and general well-being. His doctor diagnosed him with pre-diabetes. David, determined to avoid future issues, took up carb counting. "At first, it was a learning curve," he says, "but with practice, it became second nature." By measuring his carbs and adopting dietary changes, David not only improved his blood sugar control but also rekindled his passion for physical activity. "I feel like I have my energy back," he says, beaming. "Now, I can keep up with my grandkids and enjoy an active life."

Key takeaways from David's story:

Carb counting can be an effective method for avoiding blood sugar problems.

It can boost energy levels and improve general health.

With practice, carb counting can be a workable strategy for blood sugar management.

Meet Emily: Embracing a Healthy Lifestyle

Emily, a young lady with PCOS, struggled with weight control and blood sugar regulation. A registered nutritionist introduced her to carb counting, which changed her relationship with food. "I used to think healthy eating meant bland food," she said. "But carb counting allows me to explore new recipes and discover delicious options that fit my needs." Emily enjoys preparing nutritious, low-carb meals for herself and her family. "It's a win-win," she says with a smile. "We're all eating healthier and feeling better."

Key takeaways from Emily's story:

Carb counting opens the door to discovering healthy and delicious dishes.

It may be a family-friendly approach to healthy eating.

By controlling your own carbohydrate intake, you can inspire others to do the same.

These are just a handful of the many success stories related to carb counting. Remember, each trip is unique. The idea is to find a method that will allow you to take control of your health and live a fulfilling life.

Carb counting can be an effective method for controlling blood sugar levels and improving general well-being. By learning from others' experiences, adopting a positive attitude, and implementing the tactics presented in this book, you can create your own carb-counting success story and take control of your health journey.

Conclusion

Your Empowered Journey to Blood Sugar Control.

Congratulations! You've completed this comprehensive approach to blood sugar management with carb counting. This journey may appear frightening at first, but with the knowledge and tactics you've received throughout this book, you'll be well-prepared to take the thrilling path to optimal blood sugar management and a healthy you.

Remember that blood sugar management is a lifetime process, not a destination. There will be challenges and changes along the route. Accept these challenges as opportunities to learn and improve. Celebrate your accomplishments, big and small, and concentrate on the positive improvements you're making in your life.

Here's a great message to carry with you: You are not alone. There is a supportive network of people who manage their blood sugars, as well as a multitude of tools to help you.

Empower yourself with these last takeaways:

Knowledge is power. The knowledge you've received about blood sugar, carbohydrates, and carb counting allows you to make more informed diet and lifestyle decisions.

Embrace a holistic approach. Blood sugar management involves more than simply statistics. Prioritize sleep, stress management, and self-care for optimal health.

Find Your Support System: Surround yourself with positive and encouraging individuals who understand your experience.

Celebrate your successes. Recognize your achievements, no matter how minor. Celebrate progress and cultivate a positive attitude.

Believe in yourself: You can control your blood sugar and attain your health goals. Develop a growth mentality and be confident in your abilities to thrive.

This book has given you the skills and knowledge you need to start your blood sugar management journey confidently. Remember that consistency is crucial. Put your acquired information to use, adopt a healthy lifestyle, and take control of your health.

As you continue on this inspiring journey, may you experience:

Stable blood sugar levels.

Increased vigor and vitality.

Better general health and well-being.

A renewed sense of control and empowerment.

Best wishes on your exciting road toward blood sugar control!

APPENDIX

Carb content in common foods.

A comprehensive reference for the carbohydrate content of various food groups, including some hidden carb sources. Remember, serving sizes can vary, so always double-check food labels for accurate information.

Fruits (1 cup unless otherwise noted):

Apple (medium): 25 grams

Banana (medium): 23 grams

Berries (mixed): 15 grams

Cantaloupe (cubed): 11 grams

Grapefruit (half): 9 grams

Orange (medium): 15 grams

Dried fruit (raisins, 1/4 cup): 21 grams (be mindful of concentrated sugar content)

Vegetables (1 cup unless otherwise noted):

Broccoli: 5 grams

Carrots (baby): 6 grams

Green beans: 7 grams

Lettuce (mixed greens): 5 grams

Spinach: 1 gram

Tomato (medium): 5 grams

Corn (cooked): 15 grams (higher carb content compared to most vegetables)

Starchy vegetables (peas, 1/2 cup cooked): 15 grams

Grains (1 slice unless otherwise noted):

Bread (whole wheat): 16 grams

Brown rice (cooked): 22 grams

Cereal (bran flakes): 20 grams (check label for serving size)

Oatmeal (cooked): 15 grams (check label for serving size)

Whole-wheat pasta (cooked): 25 grams

Crackers (whole wheat, 3 crackers): 15 grams

Tortilla (whole wheat, medium): 20 grams

Dairy Products:

Milk (1 cup): 12 grams

Plain yogurt (Greek, 6 oz): 8 grams

Cheese (cheddar, 1 oz): 1 gram

Flavored yogurt (check label, can be high in sugar): varies

Proteins (3 oz cooked unless otherwise noted):

Chicken breast: 0 grams

Fish (salmon): 0 grams

Lean beef (ground): 0 grams

Eggs (2 large): 1 gram

Tofu (firm, 1/2 cup): 3 grams

Beans (black beans, 1/2 cup cooked): 15 grams (higher carb content)

Lentils (cooked, 1/2 cup): 18 grams (higher carb content)

Fats and Oils:

Butter (1 tbsp): 0 grams

Olive oil (1 tbsp): 0 grams

Nuts (almonds, 1 oz): 6 grams

Seeds (chia seeds, 1 tbsp): 5 grams (higher fiber content)

Snacks (Be mindful of portion sizes):

Apple slices with nut butter (2 tbsp): 20 grams (carbs from apple + nut butter)

Carrot sticks with hummus (2 tbsp): 15 grams (carbs from carrots + hummus)

Trail mix (1/4 cup): 20 grams (check label for serving size and added sugars)

Greek yogurt with berries (1/2 cup yogurt, 1/4 cup berries): 18 grams (carbs from yogurt + berries)

Hard-boiled egg: 1 gram

Edamame (shelled, 1/2 cup): 7 grams

Cottage cheese (1/2 cup): 4 grams

Hidden Carbs:

Salad dressings (check labels, can be high in sugar and carbs)

Sauces (check labels, can be high in sugar and carbs)

Breaded and fried foods (significantly higher carb content)

Processed meats (often contain added sugars and starches)

Sugar-sweetened beverages (avoid for better blood sugar control)

Tips:

Focus on whole, unprocessed foods whenever possible.

Pair carbohydrates with protein and healthy fats for balanced meals and snacks.

Read food labels carefully and pay attention to serving sizes.

Consider net carbs (total carbs minus fiber) if following a ketogenic diet (consult a healthcare professional for guidance).

This cheat sheet is a general guide. Consult a healthcare professional or registered dietitian for personalized carb counting advice.

Meal planning templates

Here are several meal plan templates to help you design a personalized carb-conscious eating routine. Remember to adjust portion sizes and carbohydrate content based on your individual needs and activity level.

Template 1

The Balanced Approach (150-200g Carbs/Day)

Breakfast (30-40g Carbs): Greek yogurt with berries and a sprinkle of granola, whole-wheat toast with scrambled eggs and avocado, oatmeal with nuts and seeds.

Lunch (50-60g Carbs): Salad with grilled chicken or fish, brown rice bowl with vegetables and lean protein, whole-wheat wrap with hummus and roasted vegetables.

Dinner (60-70g Carbs): Baked salmon with roasted vegetables and quinoa, lentil soup with a side salad, stir-fry with chicken, vegetables, and brown rice.

Snacks (2-3 Snacks with 10-20g Carbs Each): Apple slices with almond butter, handful of mixed nuts with dried cranberries, veggie sticks with Greek yogurt dip, cottage cheese with sliced cucumber and tomato.

Template 2

The Low-Carb Lifestyle (100-150g Carbs/Day)

Breakfast (10-20g Carbs): Eggs cooked to preference with spinach and cheese, chia pudding with berries and nut butter, low-carb smoothie with protein powder, avocado toast with smoked salmon.

Lunch (40-50g Carbs): Large salad with grilled chicken or steak, cauliflower rice bowl with vegetables and protein, lettuce wraps with grilled chicken or fish and low-carb dressing.

Dinner (50-60g Carbs): Grilled chicken or fish with roasted asparagus and zucchini noodles, low-carb chili with a dollop of sour cream, stuffed peppers with ground turkey and vegetables.

Snacks (2 Snacks with 5-10g Carbs Each): Celery sticks with cream cheese, olives with almonds, hard-boiled egg, small handful of berries with whipped cream.

Template 3

The High-Carb Athlete (200-250g Carbs/Day)

Breakfast (50-60g Carbs): Oatmeal with fruit and nuts, whole-wheat pancakes with berries and maple syrup, whole-wheat toast with eggs and avocado.

Lunch (60-70g Carbs): Whole-wheat pasta salad with vegetables and grilled chicken, brown rice bowl with beans, vegetables, and lean protein, whole-wheat wrap with hummus, veggies, and lean protein.

Dinner (60-80g Carbs): Baked sweet potato with grilled chicken or fish and roasted vegetables, quinoa bowl with vegetables and tofu, whole-wheat pasta with lean protein and marinara sauce.

Snacks (2-3 Snacks with 20-30g Carbs Each): Banana with peanut butter, protein bar, fruit salad with greek yogurt, whole-wheat crackers with cheese.

Template 4

The Keto-Inspired Approach (Under 50g Carbs/Day)

This template focuses on minimizing carb intake while maximizing healthy fats and protein.

Breakfast (5-10g Carbs): Scrambled eggs with cheese and spinach, keto smoothie with protein powder, almond butter, and unsweetened almond milk, chia pudding with heavy cream and berries.

Lunch (10-15g Carbs): Large salad with grilled chicken or fish, roasted vegetables with cheese, keto stir-fry with tofu, vegetables, and low-carb sauce.

Dinner (20-30g Carbs): Fatty fish like salmon or tuna with roasted Brussels sprouts, cauliflower rice with ground beef and cheese, stuffed zucchini boats with ground turkey and vegetables.

Snacks (1-2 Snacks with under 5g Carbs Each): Celery sticks with cream cheese, olives, pork rinds, small handful of nuts.

Important Note: A ketogenic diet can be restrictive and may not be suitable for everyone. Consult a healthcare professional before starting a keto diet, especially if you have any underlying health conditions.

Template 5

The Intermittent Fasting and Carb Cycling Approach

This template combines intermittent fasting (IF) windows with strategic carb cycling to optimize metabolic health.

Choose your preferred IF window: (e.g., 16:8 - fasting for 16 hours and eating within an 8-hour window).

Carb Cycling:

High-Carb Days (Post-Workout or Active Days): 150-200g carbs - Focus on complex carbs like whole grains, fruits, and starchy vegetables.

Moderate-Carb Days: 100-150g carbs - Balanced intake of complex carbs, protein, and healthy fats.

Low-Carb Days (Rest Days): 50-100g carbs - Prioritize low-carb vegetables, protein, and healthy fats.

Important Note: Intermittent fasting can be challenging for some individuals. It's crucial to listen to your body and adjust the IF window or approach if needed. Consult a healthcare professional before starting intermittent fasting, especially if you have any underlying health conditions.

Template 6

The Plant-Based Carb-Conscious Approach

This template prioritizes whole, plant-based foods while keeping an eye on carbohydrate content.

Breakfast (30-40g Carbs): Berries with chia pudding and almond milk, oatmeal with nuts and seeds, whole-wheat toast with avocado and a veggie omelet.

Lunch (40-50g Carbs): Large salad with quinoa or lentils and roasted vegetables, lentil soup with a whole-wheat roll, tofu scramble with whole-wheat toast and avocado.

Dinner (50-60g Carbs): Black bean burgers on whole-wheat buns with sweet potato fries, vegetable stir-fry with brown rice, lentil pasta with marinara sauce and vegetables.

Snacks (2-3 Snacks with 10-20g Carbs Each): Apple slices with almond butter, hummus with veggie sticks, handful of mixed nuts and dried cranberries, plant-based yogurt with berries.

Additional Tips

Rotate your protein sources throughout the week for variety and to ensure a well-rounded intake of essential nutrients.

Choose healthy fats like avocado, olive oil, and nuts to keep you satiated and support overall health.

Don't skip meals! Aim for consistent eating patterns to regulate blood sugar and prevent overeating.

Stay hydrated by drinking plenty of water throughout the day.

Consider incorporating low-carb vegetables like leafy greens, broccoli, and asparagus into your meals.

Don't be afraid to experiment and find recipes that fit your taste preferences and carb goals.

Remember: These are just templates to get you started. Customize them to your needs and preferences to create a sustainable and enjoyable carb-conscious eating routine. You can also consult a registered dietitian or healthcare professional for personalized guidance on designing a healthy carb-conscious meal plan. Feel free to mix and match elements from different templates or create your own based on your preferences and health goals. The key is to find a sustainable approach that allows you to manage your blood sugar effectively and feel your best.